ALZHEIMER'S DISEASE:
A Growing Health Care Issue
Among The Elderly

ALZHEIMER'S DISEASE:
A Growing Health Care Issue Among The Elderly

Celestina Akbar, MPA

To order additional copies of this book, contact:
Xlibris Corporation
1-888-795-4274
www.Xlibris.com
Orders@Xlibris.com
43882

Contents

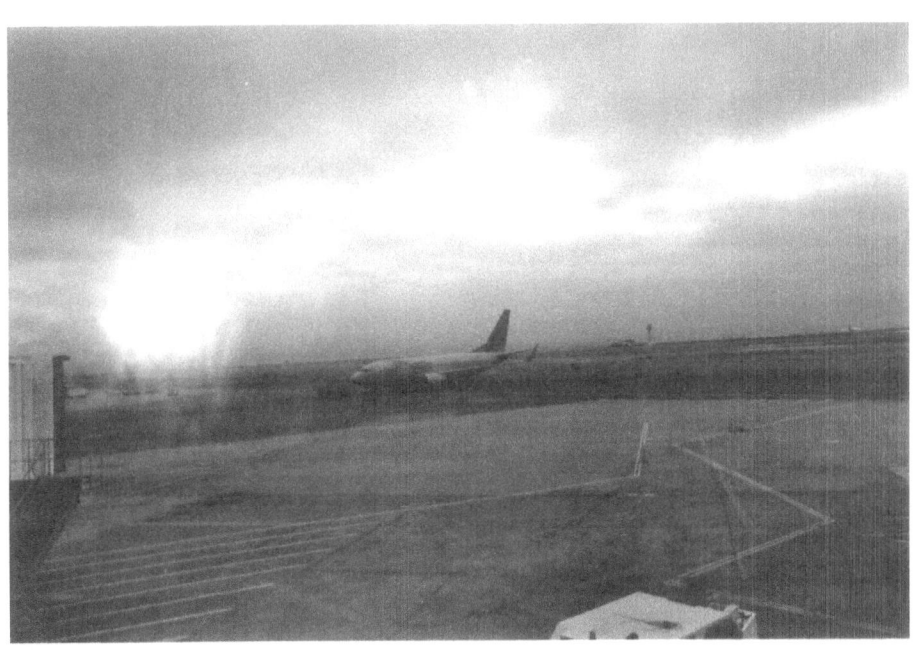

Dedicated to my widow mother, Emeline Uretha Payne.

She was a devoted, loving, caring mother to her two

children. She was afflicted with Alzheimer at the age of 86.

At age 89 she passed away to be with God.

Secondly, dedicated to former President Ronald Reagan,

who suffered from Alzheimer's disease.

Finally to the professors at Long Island University, at C.W.

Post Campus.

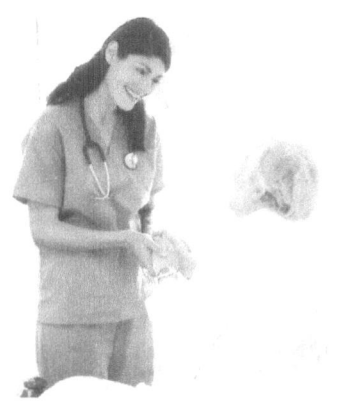

Chapter I

INTRODUCTION

Statement of the Problem

This thesis will focus on the issues surrounding Alzheimer's disease. Former President Reagan lost his battle with Alzheimer's disease during the year 2004 and reading many articles about him and this disease has been informative. According to the Alzheimer's Association (2004):

> President Reagan's legendary sense of hope and optimism were a source of inspiration to all of us, and especially to the 4.5 million Americans with Alzheimer's disease and their families and friends, and the many millions more around the globe. We are grateful that President and Mrs. Reagan worked with courage and generosity to increase public awareness of this terrible brain disease, and of the need for increased and accelerated research for effective treatments, prevention's, and a cure.[1]

Therefore, choosing this topic came from the publicity of President Reagan's stories and also because of the impact it has had on various communities and nearby surroundings of the elderly. With a declining birthrate, longer life spans, and the inevitable aging of the baby boom generation, the American population grew older throughout the 1990s.

Alzheimer's has become a significant health problem in the last 25 years because of increasing life spans and the scientific recognition that significant memory loss is not a normal part of aging. About five million elderly Americans now suffer from Alzheimer's or similar memory disorders. Most continue to live at home with the help of family, friends and paid caregivers until the late stage of the disease.

President Reagan's son spoke at the Democratic National Convention about stem cell research. It is probable that stem cell research holds out the prospect of cures for Alzheimer's, Parkinson's, cancer, and more than 70 other diseases and conditions. Newsweek (June 28, 2004) states: "in the mind of many scientists, embryonic stem cells are pulling ahead in the race toward a . . . revolution."[2]

Alzheimer's disease, the most common cause of dementia in the United States, is characterized by a slowly progressive mental deterioration. It is not only a problem for those afflicted but is also a great consequence for their families and society; since 1980 it has been the subject of intensive research. The first symptom is usually inability to remember new information. "Alzheimer's disease is extremely common, with conservative estimates of five percent of the population over age sixty-five affected. The incidence rises with increasing age, so that at least 15 to 20 percent of individuals in their eighties are affected."[3]

Alzheimer's disease is a demographic time bomb. "There are estimated to be between 10 to 20 million people afflicted with Alzheimer's world wide."[4] It is a disease primarily, but not exclusively affecting the elderly, and is typified by progressive gradual loss of memory, confusion and personality breakdown. For those who suffer from it and those who care for them, it is a very frightening disease, because early and accurate diagnosis is difficult. Alzheimer's is a very complex brain disorder. It may be better to think of it as a range of diseases with varying causes and genetic factors.

1. *The Increasing Number of People Affected by Alzheimer's is Growing*

Since 1975, the number of Americans afflicted by the disease has risen from five hundred thousand to five million. Over the next fifty years, it is estimated that between eighty and one hundred million more people worldwide will succumb to it. According to Ralph Richter, author of *Alzheimer's Disease:*

> In former times AD was regarded as a rare presenile disorder. At present, AD shows an increase in incidence and prevalence with increasing age. The incidence range in the literature from 1% to 4% of the population per year: the prevalence range from 3%

in the younger elderly (65-74 years), 19% in persons aged 75-84, up to an estimated 47% in the aged (>85 years). The prevalence of dementia increases with age. Beginning at the age of 65, every five years there is a doubling in prevalence to be expected. As women have a higher life expectancy than men, more women are expected to develop AD than men in later life.[5]

Reports in literature vary widely about the true prevalence of AD in different countries. However, there seems to be consensus "among researchers about the steadily rising number of individuals that will evidence AD over the next 30 to 40 years will probably triple." [6] Demographics study finds that 'black Americans and Hispanics may be at higher risk of developing Alzheimer's Disease than other groups."[7]

Better healthcare and technology has resulted in people living longer. Research in the field of aging and Alzheimer is accelerating at an increasingly rapid rate. Americans are witnessing a substantial increase in their elderly population more rapidly than any other nationality. In conjunction with this phenomenon comes concerns about the quality of life of persons as they age. Apparently, the Baby Boomers, are going to be the healthiest cohort of people ever to hit their 70s and 80s and probably are going to live longer than people did before. One can credit this longevity to a trend in aggressive treatments for hypertension, cholesterol, and other age-related diseases such as Alzheimer's disease. Dr. Stephen T. Dekosky, in his book, "*The Race Against an Alzheimer's Disease Epidemic*", states that: ". . . with the ability to live longer you extend the lifetime of the disease. The burden to the population will increase."[8]

2. *Definition of the Disease*

Alzheimer's disease is a progressive, irreversible brain disorder with no known cause or cure. It attacks and slowly steals the minds of its victims. Symptoms of the disease include memory loss, confusion, impaired judgment, personality changes, disorientation, and loss of language skills. It is a disease that destroys brain cells, which is not a normal part of aging.[9]

Alzheimer's is also a disease of the brain that causes a steady "decline in memory. This results in dementia, loss of intellectual functions such as thinking, remembering, and reasoning."[10]

3. *Nature of the disease and issues concerning early detection*

"If the Boomers will start to get the disease in large numbers 10 years from now, stringing these studies together end to end will probably result in us not having decent answers about prevention by the epidemic is upon us."[11] Dr. Stephen T. Dekosby elaborated on the nature and the target of prevention, observing that there is "an emphasis on early detection as well as the ability to give medications."[11]

4. *Key terms that apply to this study*

Dementia: "is an umbrella term for several symptoms related to a decline in thinking skills. Common symptoms are gradual loss of memory problems with reasoning or judgment, disorientation, and difficulty in learning. Also, other symptoms are loss of language skill and decline in the ability to perform routine tasks."[12]

Confusion: "has been defined as a mental state in which reactions to environmental stimuli are inappropriate; a state in which the person is bewildered or perplexed or unable to orientate himself."[13]

Prevalence: "is the percentage of a population that is affected with a particular disease at a given time."[14]

Baby Boomers: According to studies, these are a group of people born between 1946-1964.

The official years of the Baby Boom Generation (1946 through 1964) saw a marked increase in the number of births in North America. Here's how the birthrate rose and fell during the baby boom years:

> 1941—2,703,000 births per year
> 1946—3,311,000 births per year
> 1955—4,097,000 births per year
> 1957—4,300,000 births per year
> 1964—4,027,000 births per year

Stem cells: "Basic or primordial cells from which all human tissues and organs develop; they have the potential to differentiate, or specialize into each of the two hundred types of tissue in the body, . . . bone cells, cartilage cell, liver cells and even brain cells."[15]

Memory: "is the power or process of reproducing or recalling what has been learned and retained through associative mechanisms."[16]

Short term memory: retains up to seven items for approximately 20 seconds.

Long term memory: retain information for a longer time.

Depression "a psychiatric condition marked by sadness, inactivity, difficulty with thinking and concentration, feelings of hopelessness, and in some cases, suicidal tendencies."[17]

Caregiver: A person providing companionship and personal care to seniors in their homes including:

- Cooking and light housekeeping
- Laundry and change of bed linens
- Grocery shopping and errands
- Companionship and exercise
- Bathing, dressing and grooming assistance
- Transportation to doctor, haircuts, church
- Status reporting to family
- Hourly and live-in care available
- Help with screening for private placement
- Medication reminders

Parkinson's disease: "a disease affecting control of muscle activity, resulting in tremors, stiffness and speech impediment. In late stages, dementia can occur, including Alzheimer's disease."[17]

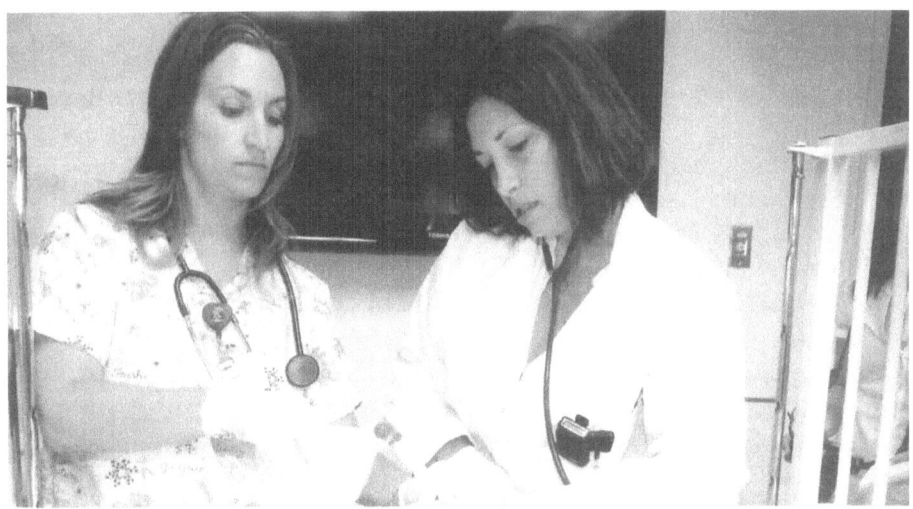

Chapter II

LITERATURE REVIEW

1. *Research conducted in the field*

Substantial literature indicates that there is no cure for Alzheimer's disease, which causes progressive dementia and eventually death. In 1995, President Ronald Reagan, in cooperation with the Alzheimer's Association, created the Ronald and Nancy Reagan Research Institute, to promote research of progress for AD. The Alzheimer's Association Reagan Research Institute is a guide committed to innovative and basic science exploring the broadest possible spectrum of approaches possible to developing Alzheimer treatments.

The goals of the Alzheimer's Association Reagan Research Institute reflect a will for successful treatments for Alzheimer's, as for other complex diseases, and will likely involve an array of strategies rather than a single magic bullet. The establishment of the Alzheimer's association, and the Reagan Research Institute is vital to research. After the Association first began awarding grants in 1982, most awards funded descriptive projects posing broad questions about the nature of Alzheimer's and its effects. Creation of the Reagan Institute helped direct evolution of the biological segment of the AD program toward funding research.

Projects in the Institute are selected by senior science staff to formulate ideas that include: processing and pathology of amyloid and other key cellular processes and pathways, genetics, animal models, inflammation and oxidative stress, and synergistic effects of vascular factors. Selected projects also represent various geographical balance and support scientists at every stage of their professional lives. In addition to funding research, the Institute also supports the activities of the Association's researchers. These teams of leaders in Alzheimer research and care, led by members of the Association's Medical and Scientific Advisory Council, provide guidance on issues in research, care giving, public policy, and programs and services.

According to a study sponsored by the Alzheimer Disease Education and Referral Center, people who have early stage Alzheimer's disease (AD) can be more capable of learning than previously thought. The promising studies suggest that "some people with early cognitive impairment can still be taught to recall important information and to better perform daily tasks."[18]

Furthermore, the study stated in a July 2004 report,

> mildly impaired AD patients who participated in three to four months of cognitive rehabilitation had a 170 percent improvement, on average, in their ability to recall faces and names and a 71 percent improvement in their ability to provide proper change for a purchase. The participants also could respond to and process information more rapidly and were better oriented. [18]

These findings, by David A. Loewenstein, Ph.D., and colleagues at the University of Miami School of Medicine and Mount Sinai Medical Center, Miami Beach, are reported in the July-August 2004 issue of the American Journal of Geriatric Psychiatry. The Loewenstein report follows a recent study by researchers at Washington University in St. Louis who found that:

> older people with early-stage AD retained functioning levels of implicit memory similar to young adults and older adults who did not have AD. Implicit memory is relatively unconscious and automatic: Information from the past pops into mind without a deliberate effort to remember. This unconscious, implicit memory is important for common skills and activities, such as speaking a language or riding a bicycle. In many cases, people implicitly remember how to perform these activities, without being able to deliberately remember when or where they learned them. The study by Cindy Lustig, Ph.D., and Randy Buckner, Ph.D., appeared in the June 10, 2004, issue of Neuron. [19]

A study prepared by Neil Buckholtz, Ph.D., head of the Dementias of Aging Branch at the NIA. Introduce

> the exciting notion that older people who are in the early stages of AD can be taught techniques to help stay engaged in everyday life," says "These findings show it is possible to pinpoint what memory capabilities are preserved in early AD and suggest ways to target those memory functions and make the most of them. [19]

Furthermore, the study indicates that,

> cognition is the ability to think, learn, and remember. Previous studies have shown that cognitive rehabilitation can effectively improve memory and other cognitive functions in people who have had strokes or suffered traumatic brain injuries. Some of these techniques also have helped improve memory in some people with AD.[19]

However, According to Neil Buckholtz, Ph.D. a current research reported by Loewenstein and colleagues is

> believed to be the first to combine several specific cognitive memory rehabilitation program for those who are mildly impaired with AD. Dr. Loewenstein and colleagues randomly assigned 44 people who were diagnosed with AD into two groups. All participants in the study were taking cholinesterase inhibitor medications, such as donepezil (Aricept), which may help prevent AD symptoms from becoming worse for a limited time.[18]

For example,

> the 25 people in the "cognitive rehabilitation" (CR) group participated in two 45-minute sessions weekly for a total of 24 sessions. During these sessions, they learned face-name recognition techniques, such as associating a prominent facial feature with a name. To enhance time and place orientation, CR participants were given memory notebooks and encouraged to record appointments, medication schedules, and contact information for relatives, friends, and doctors in them. The participants were asked to review this central information repository twice daily throughout the study.[18]

They were also taught effective ways to make change for a purchase and asked to use a calculator to balance a checkbook after paying three bills. In addition, they learned to click a mouse button in response to yellow boxes as they randomly appeared on a computer screen. This idea was designed to improve in some people. In addition, participants and their caregivers were encouraged to practice techniques that can jump start memory at home.

> The 19 participants in a "mental stimulation" (MS) group played computer games that required memory, concentration, and problem-solving skills. In addition, participants in this group were asked to discuss various topics, such as describing the neighborhood in which they grew up. They also were asked to do crossword puzzles, word scrambles, and other "homework" assignments.[18]

Furthermore,

> At the end of the study, those in the rehabilitation group showed, on average, significantly improved ability to associate faces and names, had faster mental processing speeds, were better oriented to time and place, and were better able to make correct change for purchases than those in the MS group. However, neither group showed memory improvement for manipulating objects or balancing a checkbook.[20]

A study shows that people with early AD can learn. This learning can be greatly enhanced if you teach them certain techniques that target particular areas of the brain.

> Dr. Loewenstein says., by combining specific cognitive rehabilitation strategies, we can help people with AD remain engaged in daily activities and retain a connection to their family and friends and the world as a whole for a longer period of time[20]

The June 2004 study by Lustig and Buckner recruited 34 young adults, 33 older adults without any Alzheimer's symptoms, and 24 older adults with symptoms of early-stage AD.

> The study examined a type of implicit memory that helps people act faster on items they have previously worked on than new items. In the study, participants were shown words and asked to judge if they represented something living, such as the word "DOG" or something non-living, such as the word "DESK." Overall, the

young adults made faster judgments than their older peers and those who had AD. However, all three groups were faster when shown repeated words rather than new ones. This increase was about the same for all three groups, suggesting that this benefit of implicit memory remains in old age and even early Alzheimer's disease.[20]

The researchers also used functional magnetic resonance imaging (MRI) to measure brain activity during the word judgments, which involved thinking about what words mean. Brain activity suggests rather, that seeing an item again had an important effect. Because the judgment for a word was made when the person saw it initially, the brain didn't have to work as hard at making a living/non-living judgment when the same word appeared again. In fact, even when people with AD couldn't remember which words they had seen, presenting the words again still helped them classify those words faster, and they also showed changes in brain activity like those of the young adults and their healthy older peers.

One of the exciting findings from this study is the suggestion that the brain areas supporting high level, complex thinking still have some flexibility, and these areas can change with some learning as we age and even in early AD Dr. Lustig stated that "we are hoping our results will be useful in designing cognitive training and rehabilitation programs."[21]

Another study conducted by The National Institute on Aging (NIA) in conjunction with other Federal agencies, private companies, and organizations raised approximately "$60 million, and 5-year public-private partnership . . . to test the progression of mild cognitive impairment (MCI) and early Alzheimer's disease (AD). "[22] This study could help researchers and clinicians develop new treatments and monitor their effectiveness.

> The project is the most comprehensive effort to date to find neuro imaging and other biomarkers for the cognitive changes associated with MCI and AD. Within the Federal Government, the NIA is joined in the partnership by another National Institutes of Health (NIH) Institute—the National Institute of Biomedical Imaging and Bioengineering (NIBIB)—and by the Food and Drug Administration, all of which are part of the U.S. Department of Health and Human Services. [22]

Furthermore it is important that,

> The Foundation for NIH is managing corporate, and other private participation, and has received commitments totaling more than

$20 million in contributions for the Study of Aging (ISOA), and the Alzheimer's Association. About two-thirds of the funding is expected to come from the Federal Government while private partners are expected to make up the other third. Ancillary studies will be funded by additional NIH grants. [23]

This is a vital combination of talent and resources toward a common goal—delaying or preventing Alzheimer's disease. The initiative should become a major study in the development of neuro imaging.

In April 2005, investigators will begin recruiting about 800 adults, ages 55 to 90, to participate in the research—approximately 200 cognitively normal older individuals to be followed for 3 years, 400 people with MCI to be followed for 3 years, and 200 people with early AD to be followed for 2 years.[24]

The study will compare neuro imaging, and track the progression of memory loss from its earliest stages. neuro imaging research has suggested that PET or MRI may measure more of disease progression than the neuro-psychological and cognitive assessments now typically used in research and clinical practice. As MCI and AD progress, for example, areas of the brain involved with memory, such as the hippo campus (a part of the brain heavily involved in memory) shrink using the high resolution images researchers will evaluate the best ways of measuring brain structures. Nevertheless,

previous studies have shown that low glucose metabolism can be seen in some people even before noticeable symptoms of memory loss occur. The Initiative will seek to identify additional biological factors from blood, cerebrospinal fluid (CSF), and urine samples.[25]

The important challenge is satisfaction that response to treatments will slow the progression of mild cognitive impairment and Alzheimer's disease.

For example, today, imaging is used to rule out other causes of memory problems, still not leaving the researcher or the clinician with a very clear idea of what is going on. By the end of this study, we should be able to use imaging and other biomarkers to accurately monitor disease progression and detect the effects of treatments which can slow that progression.

The NIA leads the Federal effort in research on AD and age-related cognitive change. The Institute is currently funding 6

prevention trials and 19 treatment trials for AD, in addition to
the Neuro imaging Initiative."[26]

Several promising recent developments in the study of Alzheimer's
disease may one day lead to new methods of diagnosing, preventing and
slowing the disease's progress. According to the National Institute of Health,

> "these include a new way to look inside the brains of people with
> the disease as well as new methods for preventing buildup of a
> protein, called amyloid, which forms plaques that scientists believe
> may be involved in causing Alzheimer's symptoms. Furthermore,
> detecting Alzheimer's disease at an earlier stage is a major
> research goal. In a study scientists created a compound that allows
> them to use positron emission tomography to look at early sign
> of the abnormal clumps of amylid proteins(called plaques) that
> form in the brain of people who have Alzheimer's."[27]

2. *Government resources directed to Alzheimer's disease*

There are numerous Government resources, directory and (on line)
links directed to Alzheimer's disease such as:

Medicare

Medicare is a federal health insurance program generally for people age
65 or older who are receiving Social Security retirement benefits. Medicare
covers inpatient hospital care and a portion of the doctor's fees and other
medical expenses. There are specific eligibility requirements in order for
a person to receive assistance from this program.

- Age 65 or older
- People under age 65 with certain disabilities
- People with end-stage renal disease (permanent kidney failure)

Medicare covers some, but not all, of the services a person with
Alzheimer's disease may require. Part A covers hospital. Part B covers
medical insurance

Medicare Advocacy

Alzheimer's is an epidemic that is driving Medicare costs out of control
because the program does not pay for the chronic care that could prevent

expensive but avoidable health care crises and excess disabilities. Medicare expenditures for people with Alzheimer's are nearly three times higher than the average for all beneficiaries.

> Within a decade, total annual Medicare costs for people with Alzheimer's will increase by almost 55%—to nearly $50 billion. The Medicare Advocacy Project, initiated by the Alzheimer's Association in collaboration the American Bar Association's Commission on Legal Problems of the Elderly, was developed to respond to various problems encountered by Medicare beneficiaries with Alzheimer's disease.[28]

The CMS oversees the Medicare and Medicaid programs established to combine health financing and quality assurance. Medicare is the primary health insurance program for people age 65 and older and those with certain disabilities. Medicare coverage provides acute hospital care, physician services, brief stays in skilled nursing facilities, and short-term skilled home care.

Medigap

Medicare coverage can be supplemented with Medigap, a private insurance that covers co payments and deductibles required by Medicare. The more expensive policies may cover prescription drugs.

Medicare HMO (Medicare Managed Care)

A Medicare HMO offers some additional benefits and less paperwork in exchange for restrictions on choices of hospitals, doctors, and other professionals. Most Medicare HMOs cover nursing home and home health care for limited periods only and under special circumstances.

Medicaid

Medicaid is a federal program typically administered by each state's welfare agency, and eligibility and benefits vary from state to state. The program is typically administered by a state welfare agency. Medicaid covers all or a portion of nursing home costs. A person with Alzheimer's can qualify for long-term care only if he or she has minimal income and cash assets. Medicaid covers health services for low-income individuals. People with Alzheimer's disease may receive nursing home benefits and in some States, limited community long-term care services once they meet a State' financial eligibility for Medicaid.

3. *Alzheimer Private Newsletters, Journals, Historical Literatures*

Namenda is a private series of newsletters that informs one about treating and, understanding AD providing resource library and information about caring for someone with AD. *New York City Chapter Newsletters* is published quarterly for friends and advocates in the Alzheimer's community. The mission is challenging: providing legal, financial and medical services as needed to families and support groups for caregivers. The newsletter often gives Medicaid updated information which are important to the elderly and Alzheimer's advocates, individuals, and families coping with Alzheimer's disease. November is an important month for:

> 4.5 million American suffering from Alzheimer's disease and those who care for them. In 1982, President Ronald Reagan designated November as the National Alzheimer's Disease Month. Eighteen years later, President Bill Clinton named November the National Family caregivers Month. This month provides an opportunity to recognize improvements in education, research and treatment of Alzheimer's disease.[29]

Chapter III

RESEARCH HYPOTHESIS AND METHODOLOGY

1. *Hypothesis*

1. H1: A majority of the elderly consider Alzheimer's disease as a growing healthcare issue.

   In support of my hypothesis, in our aging population, the magnitude of AD as a national health problem is steadily increasing. This makes the disease an urgent research priority. Interventions that could delay the onset of AD would have an enormous positive public health impact because they would reduce the number of people with the disease. This, in turn, would reduce the personal and financial costs associated with caring for them. A recent analysis provides a vivid illustration of the impact of delaying AD by even a few years. Moreover, this could delay Alzheimer's disease by "approximately 5 years, would reduce the numbers of persons with AD by 50 percent by the year 2050 (Brookmeyer et al., 1998)."[30]

   H2: Many middle age adults consider Alzheimer's disease as a growing healthcare issue, as it impacts on their parents and their own lives. Middle age adults consider aging is an added risk factor.

With age, the compensatory mechanisms that have evolved to cope with and eliminate free radicals become less efficient. Part of the heterogeneity of brain aging in different individuals may, in fact, be due to the generalized effect of free radicals on the brain as people age. Several ongoing clinical trials have been designed to determine whether treatment.[30]

2. *Methodology*

Describing and surveying the field. Examining attitudes of the elderly and middle age citizens, awareness of Alzheimer's disease. This will be by accomplished and reviewing previously conducted studies.

The purpose of the Alzheimer's Disease review is to understand, explain, and predict the healthcare attitudes and behaviors of people with Alzheimer's disease and their caregivers. "It is not expected that the caregiving universe is representative of the overall US population. However, there is no definitive published data on the Alzheimer's disease caregiver universe. Therefore, since it is scientifically accepted that consistent, replicable finding would indicate an accurate portrayal of the caregiver universe, the CHS caregiver sample was compared with the following studies:

> Ory, M. et al. "the Extent and Impact of Dementia Care: Unique Challenges
> Experienced by Family Caregivers. "National Institute on Aging.
> Yordi, C. et Caregiver Supports: Outcomes From the Medicare Alzheimer's
> Disease Demonstration Health Care/ financing Review (1997)
> Newman, P. et al. "Health Utilities in Alzheimer's Disease: A Cross-Sectional Study of Patients and Caregivers." Medical care (1999).
> National Family Caregivers Association 1997."[31]

Chapter IV

ANALYSIS OF WHERE WE ARE IN TREATING
ALZHEIMER'S AS A DISEASE

There are numerous centers, support groups, medical facilities, rehabilitation services and research grants available for people with Alzheimer's disease. A great number of centers support and engage in clinical and basic scientific research and promote education related to the disease. According to the Agency for Health Care Policy and Research, support groups sometimes provide consultation:

> . . . to talk things over with other people and families who are coping with Alzheimer's disease. Families and friends of people with Alzheimer's disease have formed support groups. The Alzheimer's Association has active groups across the country. Many hospitals also sponsor education programs and support groups to help patients and families.[32]

1. *Historical Analysis*

According to Manual B. Graeber, author of *Reanalysis of the First Case of Alzheimer's Disease,* the term Alzheimer's dates back to the "case record of a 51-year old female patient (Mrs. Auguste D.), who had been admitted to the Frankfurt hospital in November,1901 with signs of dementia."[33]

The article mentions that Alois Alzheimer began his medical career as assistant physician at the Municipal Hospital for Lunatics and Epileptics in Frankfurt am Main and later was promoted to 2nd physician (senior physician).

When a disease becomes as important as Alzheimer's dementia, there is a natural interest in its medical history and in the origin of the underlying disease concept, due to rapidly changing demography of an aging world. The key to understanding Alois Alzheimer's views on the disease, which was named after him, are the histological sections of the cases he saw. This histological material was rediscovered in Munich in 1992 and 1997 (Neurogenetics 1997, 1 : 73-80; 1998, 1 : 223-228).

> An extensive neuropathological and molecular genetic analysis
> of the tissue is currently being carried out. The present article
> summarizes the history of the rediscovery and provides an analysis
> of the neuropathology of Alois Alzheimer's first case, . . . [33]

Alois Alzheimer first saw Auguste D. in 1901, the first "Alzheimer patient" described in the medical literature. The clinical documentation of this case was retrieved by Maurer and colleagues in 1995 (Maurer et al., 1997).Alzheimer had moved to Munich in 1903 to build his own laboratory. Thus, when Auguste D. died in 1906, her brain was sent to him from Frankfurt as documented in the autopsy book of the Royal Psychiatric Clinic. Alzheimer presented the case of his first patient at the 37th Meeting of the Southwest German Psychiatrists in Tübingen on November 3, 1906.

Thus, this increased interest in the history of Alzheimer's disease explains why Alzheimer's cases have attracted so much attention in recent years. Dr. Alois Alzheimer headed the Anatomical Laboratory of the Royal Psychiatric Clinic in Munich from 1904 to 1912. Dr. Alzheimer published two papers on the disease which was named after him. The first report essentially represents "an abstract of the talk Alzheimer gave at the 37th Meeting of the Southwest German Psychiatrist."[33] It does not contain any identifying biographical information on the patient.

In contrast, Alois Alzheimer's second paper on the disease is a textbook-like chapter providing the clinical history as well as biographical data of another patient Alzheimer had seen at the hospital in Munich. The first name and the initial of the last name of this patient were published by Alzheimer which was common in clinical papers at the time. Thus, the information contained in Alzheimer's 1911 publication provided an excellent starting point for research. The case number of Alzheimer´s second patient, Johann F., could be identified:

> ". . . based on the autopsy book of the Psychiatric Hospital (Graeber et al., 1997; Möller and Graeber, 1998). This autopsy book was rediscovered together with other archival material in the basement of the Institute of Neuropathology of the University of Munich." [33]

Furthermore, evidence indicates that:

> Entry 784 in this autopsy book identifies a male patient bearing the last name Feigl who died on October 3, 1910, and who had been hospitalized in the Psychiatric Clinic[33]

Soon thereafter they were able to identify histological sections labeled with this same last name and the respective case number provided in the autopsy book. In addition, the admission report of the patient was found showing his first and last name and several important dates as well as matching clinical information. Interestingly, the diagnosis in the autopsy book, showed that:

> "Alzheimersche Krankheit", was written by Alzheimer himself. This was at first very puzzling to us. However, Alzheimer's boss, Emil Kraepelin, had named the disease after his co-worker in his famous psychiatry textbook which had just appeared in its eighth edition (Kraepelin, 1910). [33]

Furthermore, he thus left Alzheimer, when he made the diagnosis on Johann F., no choice but to use his own name only three years after the first description of the disease. The most likely explanation for the early acceptance of the new disease entity by Kraepelin was his personal clinical experience, i.e., seeing those cases for himself and at least some together with Alzheimer, and, importantly, the confirmatory reports that had followed Alzheimer's initial description. Kraepelin, being a scientist, stated that it appears unlikely that he" . . . based his views on anecdotal evidence, i.e., solely on Alzheimer's first report on Auguste D. It has indeed been suggested that Johann F.was the first patient to be correctly diagnosed with Alzheimer disease. [34]

This view would be in line with the fact that the autopsy report of Johann F. became part of Alzheimer's only review of the disease, which was submitted just three months after the patient's death. However, interest in the subject of Alzheimer's disease was stimulated by important field of genetics and several speculative reports suggesting that Alzheimer's first patient, August D. might have suffered from a different form of dementia.

It is believed that "Alzheimer's original patient had been affected by a rare disorder, metachromatic leukodystrophy."[35]

Nevertheless, Alzheimer's disease gained relatively rapid acceptance as a distinct disease state. In spite of this, it also gained very little attention for some decades, but has enjoyed much attention recently. In fact, it has been referred to by some as the disease of the century. Several reasons for this increased attention have been considered. Advances in both safety and medical sciences have lengthened our lives and increased the chance that any of us will suffer from maladies that tend to occur later in life. This problem is compounded by the population surge that occurred shortly after World War II. The result is an increasingly older population. As our population ages, the number of Alzheimer patients "could triple to 14 million, or about one in twenty Americans."[36]

Additionally, people don't die directly from Alzheimer's disease but from complications such as pneumonia to which their level of incapacitation at advanced stages of the disease make them susceptible. In earlier decades of this century, a cause of death would more likely have been listed as pneumonia, whereas now, with increased awareness, and therefore diagnosis of Alzheimer's, the primary disease is more likely to be listed as the cause of death.

As we begin the 21st century we are seeing an overwhelming increase in dementia illnesses. According to Dr. David Perlmutter, a Neurologist at present:

> ". . . approximately 4.5 million American have Alzheimer's disease. By the year 2030 it has been estimated that this number will approach 9 million. Alzheimer's disease has been estimated to be 50% in individuals 85 years or older the most rapidly growing segment of our population."[37]

Early Efforts

Prior studies about early onset of Alzheimer's disease were prepared in Scotland, and focused not only on familial factors but rather on environmental factors as well. Geographical differences in countries between urban and rural areas and within a single large city posed many questions in AD about exposure to harmful environmental factors and the relation to AD.

However, the disease was first described by Dr. Alois Alzheimer in 1906. Since then, researchers have developed a deeper understanding of the changes in the brain (plaques and tangles) and behavioral changes that characterize the disease. Identifying risk factors are age and family history.

Most people diagnosed with Alzheimer's disease are older than age 65; however, many can be diagnosed in their 40s or 50s.

Policy/Programs

The public policy of the Alzheimer's Association is based on the commitment to support persons with Alzheimer's disease or a related disorder and their caregivers throughout the progression of their disease and to help promote prevention and /or a cure for the disease. For this reason, the Alzheimer's organization has stated that they are ". . . committed to public policy efforts that provide quality care throughout the long term care continuum. Specifically, . . . promoting efforts . . long term care environments for caregivers . . ."[38]

2.   Financial Analysis of Impacts of the Disease

Managing finances for people with Alzheimer's is a balancing act. Whether it's simply balancing a checkbook or weighing the pros and cons of an investment strategy, the ability to confidently handle finances requires sound thinking abilities and judgment. In general, for people in the early stages of Alzheimer's disease, financial abilities are often the first functional life skills to deteriorate.

According to a recent report from the Family Relief Program, the total cost for the care and treatment of the victims of Alzheimer's disease nationwide has reached over "$100 billion annually."[39] In addition Alzheimer's patient caring services at home:

> ". . . between $18,000 and $20,000 per year. According to a survey conducted in 2003 by General Electric Financial, the annual cost for nursing home care in the U.S. ranges from $35,900 to $166,700, with the average being $57,700."[40]

Early-onset Alzheimer's can pose unique challenges for the patient and their family. You may still be working outside the home, but your symptoms may cause you to retire early and possibly lose income and insurance benefits. They and their family need to plan and to prepare for financial challenges. They should know some basic information on how to handle your finances while living with Alzheimer's disease. There are professional financial managers and medical lawyers who deal with financial planning for people with long-term or progressive illnesses.

It is important to consider financing options. Long-term financial planning is important for everyone but is essential if they are coping with the expense of a long-term illness, such as Alzheimer's disease. Many people pay careful attention to their health after they are diagnosed with Alzheimer's. They research their treatment plan, take their medications on schedule, and consult with their physician regularly. However, it may take some time for patients and caregivers to realize that a progressive illness like Alzheimer's can have a tremendous effect on their financial well-being. The Alzheimer's Association may be able to give a list of insurers with a high level of Alzheimer's coverage. People that are 65 or over, may qualify for Medicare. "Medigap policy, which is a supplement insurance that is available through a private insurer. Also that many states have prescription assistance/reimbursement programs for low-income senior citizens."[41] If they are disabled but too young to qualify for Social Security, they may be eligible to receive a form of Medicare for the disabled. If they cannot get insurance and their income is low they may qualify for Medicaid, a government safety net program that pays for medical costs that exceed a person's ability to pay. If they are too young to qualify for Social Security, they should consider state-run disability programs, unless they are enrolled in their employer's disability coverage. "If their total income is below a certain level, they may qualify for federally subsidized supplemental Security income"[42]

With an Alzheimer's diagnosis often comes a new financial demand required to maintain care both within the home and outside the home. To ensure that adequate finances will be available, families must consider evaluating the following expenses, such as doctor visits, prescription, and housing both now and in the future. It is essential that current sources of income, including personal savings, investment, employee or retirement benefits, and insurance are evaluated. Other "financial resources are available, through government organization."[43]

The following are recommendations for persons afflicted with Alzheimer's. You should evaluate current financial situation, of the person with Alzheimer's disease.

- Trying to anticipate the additional expenses as the disease progresses.
- Considering hiring a qualified financial advisor.
- Doing what can now to prepare for the financial challenges that may await you later.[44]

3. *Government Resources for Alzheimer's Families*

Health insurance can play a key role in helping to ease some of the financial burden on long term care. The most common form of insurance includes Medicaid and Medicare, which are both provided by the government.

Medicaid is a federal program whose eligibility and benefits vary by state. The program is typically administered by a state welfare agency. Medicaid covers all or a portion of nursing home costs A person with Alzheimer's disease can qualify to receive long-term care only if he or she has minimal income and cash assets.

Medicare is the major government program for health care financing in the United States. It is universal based on age and or permanent disabilities of the enrollees. Its financing and administration is entirely federal and thus the program may vary from state to state. For example,

> With deductibles and coinsurance, it covers the cost of inpatient hospital care and physician's services. It also covers a limited number of nursing home days for people judged to have rehabilitation potential and who require skilled care.[45]

4. *Non Profit, Resources for Alzheimer's Families*

There are numerous resources from non-profit organizations that are receiving grants to provide services and guidance to people afflicted with Alzheimer's disease such as:

FamiliesUSA: The Voice for Health Care Consumers is a national, non-profit, non-partisan organization dedicated to promoting high quality, affordable health care and long term care. Act as a watchdog over government actions affecting health care, alerting consumers to changes and helping them have a say in the development of policy. Produce highly respected health policy reports describing the problems facing health care consumers and outlining steps to solve them.

American Association Of Retired Persons provides useful information and product discounts for those over 50."[46] Membership would aim to encourage, rather than coerce family members into taking greater responsibility for dementing and dependent elderly relatives with tax incentives that will yield stronger encouragement.

5. *Social Analysis*

The following quality of data was reveal from one study that:

> Alzheimer's Disease afflicts 3% of persons aged 65 to 74.
> Alzheimer's Disease afflicts 18.7% of persons aged 75 to 84.
> Alzheimer's Disease afflicts 47.2% of persons aged 85 and over.
> Alzheimer's Disease is more prevalent in females than in males.[47]

With population trends skewing toward a larger percentage of elderly, (see page 25 for discussion of population) Alzheimer's disease is projected to afflict many millions in the United States and around the world in the future. In terms of cost and psychological burden, the anticipated burden of this disease on caregivers and society at large is staggering.

We are learning more about how the brain is affected in Alzheimer's. We do not yet know how to prevent or cure it. But we do know how to treat its symptoms. Aricept® is a drug that has been shown to help treat the symptoms of mild to moderate Alzheimer's. Mild stage symptoms are "memory loss, forgetting names of common household items, say the same things over and over, loses things very often, need more support to be independent."[48]

There are two additional stages as the disease progresses. The moderate stage, whose which symptoms include "poor memory of recent events, forgets to shave or shower, argue often"[49] and severe stages include inability to speak words clearly, and dependency on a caregiver for all needs.

Geographical and Social analysis of Population affected by the Problem

The main risk factor for Alzheimer's disease is increased age. The rates of the disease increase markedly with advancing age, because about 25 percent of people over 85 suffering from Alzheimer's or other severe dementia. Some investigators, describing a family pattern of Alzheimer's disease, suggest that in some cases, heredity may influence its development. A genetic basis has been identified through the discovery of "several genetic markers on chromosomes 21 and 14 for a small subgroup of families in which the disease has frequently occurred at relatively early ages." [50]

Some evidence points to chromosomes as implicated in certain other families that have frequently had the disease develop at later ages. At the same time, data indicate that the likelihood that a close relative of an afflicted individual will develop Alzheimer's disease is low. In most cases, such an individual's risk is only slightly higher than that of someone in the general population, where the lifetime risk is below one percent. And, of course, many disorders have a genetic potential that is never expressed—that is, despite being at risk for a certain illness, one might go through life without ever developing any symptom of the disease. Nevertheless, an adult population studied with AD diagnosed on the basis of standardized criteria of the "*Diagnostic and Statistical Manual of Mental Disorders,* 4th edition . . . Treatment included therapeutic doses for at least 12 weeks."[51]

According to a Canadian Study of Health and Aging,

> One in 20 Canadians over age 65 has AD. Thus, in 2001 an estimated 238, 000 Canadians over 65 had AD, and 60 000 new cases were expected per year. The Canadian Consensus Conference on Dementia and others recommend cholinesterase inhibitors for standard symptomatic treatment of AD. [52]

According to Canadian census, the population grew between "1996 and 2001, by four per cent, to 30,007,094 inhabitants. The national median age—the age where half the population is older and half is younger—rose from 35.3 in 1966 to 37.6 in 2001."[53]

Few diseases affect more Americans, require more prolonged treatment, cause more suffering for the families of the afflicted, and waste more precious human financial resources then Alzheimer's disease. "An estimated 4 million persons suffer from Alzheimer's, or about one in 10 Americans over age 65 and nearly half of those over age 85."[54]

As the baby boom generation shoulders its way into old age, few diseases represent a greater threat to the health and financial well being of society as whole. Within the next few decades, "14 million individuals will be stricken with Alzheimer's, raising the annual cost of caring for its victims to $375,000,000.[55]

Because of its critical size and tragic impact, Alzheimer's disease represents one of the nation's most vexing health problems. After two decades of intensive research, scientists have begun to understand the basic mechanisms of Alzheimer's as well as the complex interplay of genetic and environmental risk factors. But if society hopes to avert widespread suffering and enormous strain on its health care system, science must act now because "researchers believe that Alzheimer's actually begins 10 to 20 years before its first symptoms appear."[56]

Studies that have been conducted

According to Lawrence Whalley, author, of British Journal of Psychiatry, informative, community based studies aims to integrate recent studies on genetic and environmental factors in AD into a "multi-factorial disease model."[57]

Moreover, the British Journal of Psychiatry stated that:

> ". . . genetic epidemiology of AD are rare. Putative risk factors from the Scottish studies include increased paternal age in AD men

and coal mining as paternal occupation in both AD and vascular
dementia. migration effects suggest that environmental factors
in high incidence AD areas are important during adult life." [57]

"Drugs can reverse symptoms by several months but cannot slow the
progress of neuron degeneration."[58] Certain natural supplements taken
in combination with and without prescription medication may reduce the
likelihood of the disease or delay its onset or slow its progress.

There are many experimental approaches to treating Alzheimer's
disease, including the vaccine, trying to prevent the further formation
of amyloid plaques, or removing some of them from the brain. But, Dr.
Morgan said, by the time memory loss becomes apparent, the toxic plaques
are probably accumulating too quickly to eliminate enough amyloid
needed to restore normal memory. A study from Angelfire.suggests a new
approach to treating this disease that would enhance ". . therapy to reduce
the amyloid load and then start the patient on a memory-enhancing drug
to block the effect of any remaining amyloid on normal learning and
memory." [59]

Social cost

As medical research continues to bring forth significant discoveries
related to Alzheimer's, that bring us to a deeper understanding of the
disease processes, social research can bring us closer to understanding
more completely the human and economic costs of the disease. The
business sector of the American economy contributes mightily to the
nation's expenditures related to Alzheimer's. According to an article in
U.S. Business Reports, the combined total cost to businesses of Alzheimer's
disease is:

> more than $33 billion. And, as Dr. Koppel points out, many of the
> costs associated with the disease could not be measured within
> this study, so that the actual cost of the disease—both to society
> and to businesses—is far greater than projected[60]

Goals of the social policy

The goals of the social policy is to have all resources of expanded
coverage for community based long-term care in two important ways:

> By documenting the extent to which non-institutionalized
> long-term care patients rely on the assistance of family members

and friends, and by evaluating the effect of this assistance on the utilization of outpatient rehabilitative and personal care services.[61]

6. *Political Analysis—Developing of Legislation*

While AD remains a mystery with its cause and cure not yet discovered, there is considerable excitement and hope about new findings that are unfolding in numerous research settings. The connecting pieces to the puzzle called Alzheimer's disease continue to be found. There are more and more partners involved in the effort, with growing national interest. For instance:

> The Clinton Administration has designated $50, million to be used over five years for research in to Alzheimer's disease, an ailment that disrupts thinking, memory and language skills among the elderly.[62]

At the same time, federal, state, community, corporate, and foundation support for new studies and better services are all on the rise:

> The administration's announcement . . . coincided with new coming out of the first World Alzheimer Congress 2000 in Washington that a possible vaccine against the disease has passed safety trials.[62]

The U.S. Department of Health and Human Services established a Department Task Force on Alzheimer's Disease. This task force "legislatively mandated as the Council on Alzheimer's Disease."[63] In addition, a non-federal advisory panel on Alzheimer's disease was established by congressional action.

> The panel, which works closely with the Council, consists of 15 national authorities on Alzheimer's disease selected for their depth and breadth of expertise in this area[63]

The work of both the Council and the Panel reflect the concern and interest that is being focused by the federal government on Alzheimer's disease. The result recommended by the Council on Alzheimer's were to:

1. Sustain a coordinated focus on genetics and public health at CDC.
2. Establish mechanisms for external input, particularly for ethical, legal, and social issues.

3. Provide public health professionals with training opportunities to enhance their skills and knowledge.
4. Develop a strategy for communication about genetics[64].

The U.S. health care system is currently undergoing two major transformations. First, public programs in health and social services are being reorganized, downsized, and privatized. "These changes are reshaping and redefining the responsibility for social welfare programs that have provided health and income support for poor, elderly, and disabled persons for decades."[65] Second, even more dramatic changes are taking place in the private health care market. These include the shift to managed care, increasing vertical and horizontal integration, and the forging of new relationships among insurers, providers, and purchasers in an increasingly competitive market.

These agencies and organizations also will be expected to support and conduct research and evaluations to assess how well the market is meeting critical health care objectives and how well they then disseminating the findings of their research. In particular, it will be important to have objective, scientific answers to questions in these areas:

> Effects of changes on the capacity of public programs and the private health care market. Extent to which these social experiments result in the anticipated individual behavior (e.g., will Medicaid beneficiaries decrease use of emergency services?). [57]

Current Political Aspects of Stem Cell Research

Stem cell research holds out the prospect of a cure for Alzheimer's, as well as other diseases, such as Parkinson's. There is possibility that a cure is out there and yet, because of President Bush's edict, in 2001, it is very hard to accept that the cure may be delayed or not reached at all. According to the Washington Post, Michael Reagan, spoke out about stem cell research at the Democratic Convention. He spoke on the need to lift restrictions that limit federally funded research to stem cell. According to researchers, stem cell research may offer promising avenues for the future treatment or cure of some dementia, such as Alzheimer's disease.

The Alzheimer's Association of Australia, stated that ". . . the involvement of scientist and agencies in all aspects of stem cell research in Australia will promote the best access for Australians with dementia to any treatment that may result from research."[66] However, the recommendations of the Australian's House of Representatives Standing Committee on Legal and Constitutional Affairs provide a solid basis to support and manage stem cell research in Australia. While there may be important potential for new treatment through, "embryonic research, work in this area should be closely regulated, avoiding any possibility of the deliberate creation of embryos for research purposes."[66]

The Clinton Administration published guidelines governing the use of "human embryonic stem cells in the Federal Register on August 23, 2000. On April 25, 2001, a scheduled review of pending grant applications was postponed to provide President George W. Bush and his new Administration an opportunity to review the issue."[67] On August 9, 2001, President Bush issued a long-awaited decision on stem cell research. He authorized funding of stem cell research using existing pluripotent stem cell lines that were derived from human embryos before August 9. Such research is eligible for federal funding if the following criteria are met:

1) there must have been informed consent of the donors, 2) the embryos must have been created for reproductive purposes and in excess of clinical need, 3) there must not have been any financial inducements to the donors, and 4) the embryos must not have been created for research purposes.[67]

During the fiscal year 2002, the National Institute of Health (NIH) funded the first grants to conduct human embryonic stem cell research, including both new grants and supplements to existing grants. Many people believe stem cell related cures for hard-to-treat illnesses like Parkinson's and Alzheimer's are just a few years off. The truth, Michael Reagan says, is that such cellular therapies are decades away. Moreover, he adds, "it's not that stem cells themselves, per se, will be the cure. It's that in figuring out how stem cells work, we're getting at fundamental aspects of the body."[68] So while stem cell research is a bonanza for basic biological knowledge, clinical applications are likely to be a long way off.

The media continues to report that the family of former President Reagan are in favor of stem cell research. Former President Reagan's suffering under Alzheimer's disease was tragic, and we should do everything we can that is ethically proper to help others afflicted with it. According to his son, Michael Reagan:

". . . urged our nation to look to adult stem cell research—which has yielded many clinical successes—and away from the destruction of developing human lives, which has yielded none.[69]

Furthermore, the media warned, "Those who would trade on Ronald Reagan's legacy should first consider his own words." [69] Researchers have apparently known for some time that embryonic stem cells will not be an effective treatment for Alzheimer's, because as two researchers told a Senate subcommittee in May, 2004 it is a:'whole brain disease,' rather than a cellular disorder such as Parkinson's. This has generally been kept out of the news. Stem cell experts confess . . . that of all the diseases that may be someday cured by embryonic stem cell treatments, Alzheimer's is among the least likely to benefit.[69]

Current Proposals for Policy-Initiatives

Federal:

It was reported by the Associated Press at Newsday.com. that Senator Hillary Rodham Clinton wanted to create a nationwide electronic medical system that would enable doctors to access and share health records, research, prescriptions and other information. She also envisions patients accessing lab results online, recording daily blood sugar levels in their electronic record, receiving prompts to take their medication and communicating more often with doctors by e-mail. Clinton (D-NY) told about 100 New York City health care leaders at Manhattan's New York-Presbyterian Hospital

> "But the systems are not usually in place to do any of that, and these barriers to communication don't serve physicians and they don't serve patients and they are not good for our country.".[70]

The federal initiatives are needed: HIPAA, Standardized Code Set, E-HIM (Electronic Health Information Management) with full, authorized access for patients, providers, and carriers. The results, according to a study by the physician-led Center for Information Technology Leadership, a fully functional national system of healthcare information . . . will generate a net value of up to "$77.8 billion a year in savings over costs. The report entitled The Value of Health Care Information Exchange and Interoperability was published online by the policy journal Health Affair."[70]

State Efforts:

The proposed legislative agenda for the Maine Alzheimer's Association is based on the commitment to support a person with Alzheimer's disease. Commitment to public policy efforts that provide quality care throughout the long-term care are essential. Specifically, the Maine Alzheimer's Association supports the availability of home and community based services.

> Seventy percent of all people with Alzheimer's disease, or their families care for related disorders at home. Since the disease can take from three to more than twenty years to run its course, families are often unable to afford the help they need over a long period of time.[71]

The main Alzheimer's Association believes that workforce issues should be a policy priority. "Direct care staff has been identified as a key to quality care we support continued legislative attention to the crisis in the long-term care workforce."[71] Other broad—based policy initiatives that the Association monitors include:

> Support for ongoing and emerging initiatives that will assist elders in purchasing, needed prescription medication, protect against the abuse and exploitation of persons with Alzheimer's disease and monitor consumer rights issues."[71]

The California Stem Cell Research and Cures Initiative, announced the measure has been endorsed by the Alzheimer's Association California Council. The initiative, which will appeared on the November, 2004 ballot, would provide funds needed for the development of lifesaving therapies and cures for diseases that could save the lives of millions of California children and adults and reduce health care costs.

The Alzheimer's Association joins a growing coalition of grassroots supporters such as: Nobel prize-winning scientists and medical experts, families involved in patient advocacy and efforts to cure diseases, and organizations like the California Medical Association, American Nurses Association of California, American Diabetes Association, Christopher Reeve Paralysis Foundation, Juvenile Diabetes Research Foundation, Elizabeth Glaser Pediatric AIDS Foundation, Sickle Cell Disease Foundation of California, ALS Therapy Development Foundation, Parkinson's Action Network, the California Congress of Seniors, the Gray Panthers, and the National Coalition for Cancer Research.

Foundations Efforts

According to Census 2000, 12.5 percent of the US population is hispanic/latino, and this population increased 58 percent between 1990 and 2000. As the hispanic/latino population grows, it will increasingly face Alzheimer's disease. "Accessing healthcare resources is affected by cultural attitudes and practices. Therefore, it is important to create culturally appropriate educational materials and programs that competently and accurately communicate with spanish-speaking persons,"[72] said Kathleen O'Brien, senior vice president, program and community services, Alzheimer's Association. Alzheimer's disease knows no boundaries—people of all races and ethnicity are affected. Yet, unfortunately, many minority groups in the United States encounter obstacles that limit their access to information, care and health resources.

To help the Alzheimer's Association reach out to the hispanic/latino community,

> MetLife Foundation has made a $175,000 grant to fund the development of guides and brochures in Spanish. As well as provide support to the Association's nationwide chapter network across the United States for local outreach activities to Hispanic/Latino communities. [73]

The National Endowment for Alzheimer's Research (NEAR) was established in 2001 as a public charity. Their major sponsors are "Apple Computer, International Scientific Publications, Staples, The Home Depot, The Publications Group, Inc. and Work Life Matters."[74] Furthermore, according to National Foundation Sources, the following represents more nonprofit foundation that fund programs related to the aging, mental, and Alzheimer's disease:

- AARP Andrus Foundation: It supports four areas research, innovations, research of information, training the next generation of researchers in aging.
- Archstone Foundation: supports professional training programs for those preparing for a career in gerontology
- Alzheimer's Association: support ongoing research or pilot projects related to Alzheimer's disease and related disorders.
- Brookdale Foundation: focuses on needs and challenges of America's elderly, respite service for people with Alzheimer's disease.
- "The John A. Hartford Foundation: seek to enhance academic Geriatrics and Training, and Integrating and Improving Services for Elders.
- Robert Wood Johnson Foundation: is the largest U.S. foundation contributing to health care programs."[75]

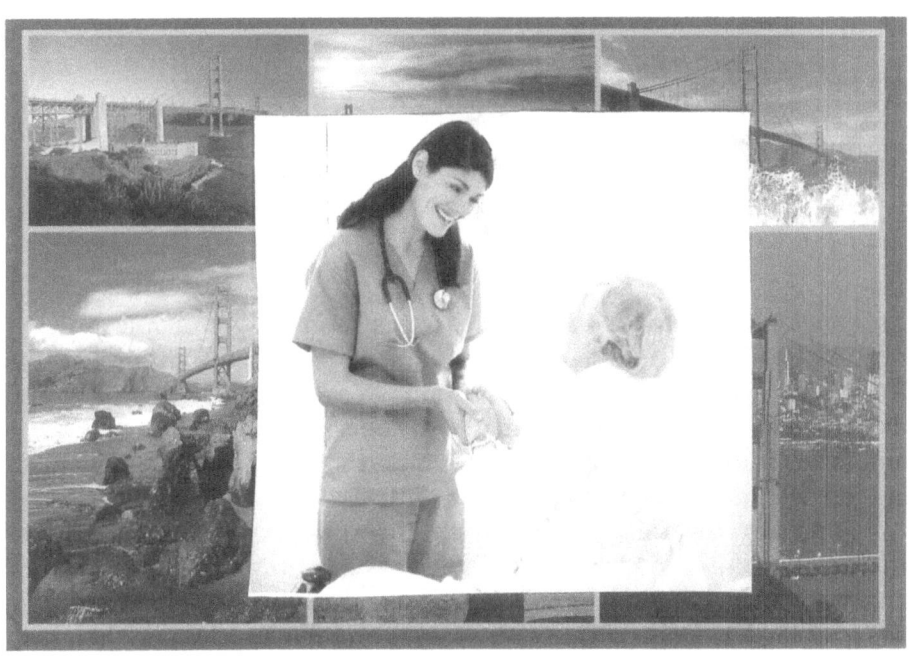

Chapter V

CONCLUSIONS

This book has highlighted significant issues and needs of people afflicted with Alzheimer's disease and the understanding of the occurrence of AD. Many studies, services and programs were reviewed concerning the diagnostic work up of patients with the Alzheimer's disease. Hopefully, these and other studies will help future researchers to disentangle the genetic and environmental factors associated with AD.

There are several reasons why the hypotheses: "H1: A majority of the elderly consider Alzheimer's disease as a growing healthcare issue" approves, and "H2: Many middle age adults consider Alzheimer's disease as a growing health care issue, as it impacts on their parents and their own lives" expresses approbation.

First, these hypotheses test that the incidence of Alzheimer's disease is increasing at an alarming rate along with the aging of our population. The vast majority of Alzheimer's disease is acquired or classified by unknown cause of conventional medicine. There is much discussion about the cause of Alzheimer's disease and many consider that a single agent may not cause Alzheimer's disease.

Second, these hypotheses reveal based on research, that Alzheimer's disease is the leading cause of dementia in the elderly and is the fourth leading cause of death in developed nations after heart disease, cancer, and stroke. More often dementia cases are due to Alzheimer's disease, with blood vessel disease and stroke being the second most common causes.

Third, as stated in Chapter 1, page 6 as age advances, the risk of developing Alzheimer's disease rises sharply. The frequency of Alzheimer's among 60-year-olds is about 1%. This incidence doubles approximately every 5 years, becoming 2% at age 65, 4% at 70, 8% at 75, 16% at 80, and 32% at 85. It is estimated that as many as two-thirds of those in their nineties suffer from some form of dementia. For those who aspire to live a very long life, dementia is a threat second only to death. Some believe that dementia is a natural way to end life.

Fourth, there are over 100,000 deaths per year related to Alzheimer's disease. Four million people and their families suffer from this disease. Annual costs to the United States from Alzheimer's disease are over $60 billion. If a treatment was developed that only delayed the onset of the disease by five years, costs to society would decrease by about half and save $30-$40 billion each year in this country alone (Chapter II, page 20).

Also, one in ten Americans over 65 and nearly half of those over age 85 do suffer from Alzheimer's. On the other hand, in Canada, one in 20 Canadians over age 65 has AD. This indicates that more Americans have a greater threat to health and well being. In addition, the elderly should be aware that the annual Medicare spending for beneficiaries with AD will "grow four-fold by 2025 to $294 billion, and will be over $1 trillion by 2050. Medicaid spending on persons with AD will reach $32 billion by 2025 and $118 billion by 2050."[76] If we can delay the onset of Alzheimer's or slow its progression, savings to Medicare and Medicaid will be enormous. Moreover, these hypotheses will encourage discussion about:

- What has been the elderly's most profound Alzheimer—related life change?
- What sources do middle age people have or need to cope with this change?
- What is the elderly most critical practical concern about having Alzheimer's or caring for someone with it?
- What is the elderly most important emotional concern about having the disease, or caring for some one with it?
- What questions do the elderly still have about Alzheimer's?
- Do others have questions or can they recommend resources?
- What resources have the elderly have found resourceful?

Recommendations for Policy

In the fall of 2003, material published did not recommend that healthy people under age 50 get the flu vaccine. Adults should be concerned about the risk they themselves accumulate by taking the vaccine each year. If an individual had five flu shots between 1970 and 1980, the chances of getting Alzheimer's disease are ten times higher than a person who had fewer shots."[77] Policy recommendations include:

1) Provide additional education, and training opportunities to providers, and caregivers.
2) Provide adequate financial assistance to those who cannot afford the high cost of nursing home care.
3) Ensure that persons with Alzheimer's disease are not discriminated.[77]

As indicated in Chapters II, III, and IV, the following are recommendations across a variety of policy domains related to Alzheimer's disease as follows:

- First, according to chapter IV, page 48, the U.S. Office of the Aging and the U.S. Office of the Attorney General, in conjunction with the Advisory Council on Quality Care at the End of Life, the Alzheimer's Association, and other interested groups, should develop a guide for serving as a health care proxy for a patient with AD.
- Second, based on federal initiatives stated on page 47, the General Assembly in Washington should amend the Health Care Decisions Act to clarify the circumstances under which research participation is encompassed by the Act's definition of health care.
- Third, based on research, conducted, Chapter II, U.S. Office of Aging and Human Services and local agencies and departments of Health and Human Services should consider whether additional continuing education or other efforts are appropriate to improve end-of-life decision making on behalf of wards with AD.
- Fourth, according to state initiatives, in Chapter IV, the New York Advisory Council on Quality Care at the End of Life should review the directive forms and consider whether a single, optional form that encourages the designation of a health care agent should replace the two forms now set out in the Health Care Decisions Act and whether the materials accompanying the form should encourage the informal expression of preferences and values, rather than instructions about specific life-sustaining medical treatments.
- Fifth, based on other broad initiative mentioned in Chapters III and IV, the New York Advisory Council on Quality Care at the End of Life should review health care facilities.
- Sixth, in support of the hypotheses in Chapter III and various foundation efforts, the New York Advisory Council on Quality Care at the End of Life should consider how advance directives

and other tools of advance care planning can most effectively be made available to cultural and linguistic minority groups. As a first step, consideration should be given to translating advance directive forms and related materials into Spanish.

- Seven, based on electronic health information, the Health Policy Division of the U.S. Office of the Aging, should explore the feasibility of an empirical study of research advance directives, with the goal of basing future policy recommendations on the data analysis.

- Eight, according to federal initiatives described in chapter IV, the U.S. General Assembly should enact legislation requiring preprinted durable power of attorney forms (other than those used by lawyers or financial institutions under circumstances that allow for personal explanation of the document's significance) to contain a plainly worded disclosure about the effect of executing the document.

- Ninth, based on literature review, in Chapter II, the federal Medicaid Program should take steps to assure that its participating managed care and peer review organizations do not deem a service to be medically unnecessary or inappropriate for a patient based solely on the fact that the patient has been diagnosed with AD.

- Tenth, according to Chapter II, the federal Medicaid Program should take appropriate steps to revise the level of care assessment tool as promptly as possible and work in collaboration with the Alzheimer's Association to enhance the sensitivity of the tool for AD patients.

- Eleventh, the federal Medicaid Program should promptly review whether Transmittal 135 has outlived its usefulness and should be replaced.

- Twelfth, according to methodology discussed in Chapter III, official of the federal Medicaid Program should consult with representatives of nursing homes and hospices to consider how to remove financial disincentives to the use of hospice in nursing homes.

- Thirteenth, according to electronic health information stated on page 47, surveyors from the Office of Health Care Quality should be provided with suitable training regarding the use of feeding tubes for patients with AD, including the clinical indications and legal criteria justifying the withholding or withdrawal of a feeding tube.

- Fourteenth, the Office of Health Care Quality should continue to emphasize to its licensees that its surveys will give priority attention to evidence of appropriate pain assessment and management and train its surveyors to be particularly vigilant about this aspect of quality care.

- Fifteenth, according to Chapter III, the associations representing nursing homes should give priority to educational efforts to convey best the practices in pain assessment and management, with particular emphasis on tools that permit pain in people with AD to be measured and documented (by, for example, consistent observation of well-defined aspects of breathing, vocalization, facial expression, and body language).
- Sixteenth, as resources permit, the Office of Health Care Quality should conduct or sponsor a study to determine whether advertising claims about special AD care are consistent with descriptions in disclosure statements and whether both are consistent with services actually delivered.
- Seventeenth, based on historical analysis Chapter IV, on page 31, the U.S. Office of Aging should convene a meeting of interested parties to begin the process of identifying, pilot testing, and promoting a well-designed and validated abuse prevention program in nursing homes and assisted living facilities.
- Eighteenth, as stated in chapter IV, the U.S. Department of Health and of Human Services should work with interested groups to consider the need for improved services to victims of dementia-related domestic violence and the individuals with AD who have acted violently as a consequence of their disease and increase awareness of the risk posed by an AD patient's having access to firearms in the home and the safety measures that might be taken.
- Nineteenth, in support of growing coalition of grassroots supporters, page 49, the U.S. General Assembly should prohibit discrimination in access to long term care insurance based on genetic profile.

In summary, I learned through this project that both environmental and genetic factors are associated with AD. I also found that many organizations, hospitals, and researchers are working to help the elderly afflicted with AD because Alzheimer's disease is the leading cause of dementia in the elderly and is the fourth leading cause of death after heart disease, cancer and stroke.

References

Alzheimer's Association Australia (Mar., 02) *Policy Position on Stem Cells.* Retrieved Dec. 12, 2004 from *http://www.alzvic.asn.au/stemcells.htm*

Associated Press and Reuters (2000, July 16). CNN on the web. pages 1-4 Retrieved Dec 9,2004, from *http//archives.cnn.com*

Bensing, Karen McNally "Forgetting to remember" [on line] Available: *http://web7.infotrac.galegroup.com/itw/infomark/662/529/49538996w7/*

Biotech web site from *www.biotechanalyticas.com/Topics/alzheimers.htm*

Cohen, Richard 2004 *The Washington Post:* Ron Reagan [on line] Available: *http://proquest.umi.com/*

Consumer Health Science (2004) *Methodologies* Retrieved Nov.15, 2004: *www.chsinternational.com/methodology_alzheimers_caregiver_project.asp*

Dekosby, Stephen T., M. D. (2001) *The Race Against an Alzheimer Disease Epidemic* (as cited on line) available: *www.alz.org/internationalconference/pressreleases/ 71804_awards.asp*

Filten, L.J. & Vellas, B. (2001) *Research and Practice in Alzheimer's Disease.* New York: Springer Publishing Co.

Gauthier, Serge & Cummings, *Jeffrey L M.D.(2002) Alzheimer's Disease and Related Disorders Annual2002,* Martin Dunitz Publisher Ltd.

Gilhooly, Mary L.(1986) *The Dementias, Policy and Management. New Jersey: Prentice Hall*

Gray-Davidson, Frena (1999) *The Alzheimer's Sourcebook fir Caregivers* Los Angeles : NTC Contemporary Publishing Group

Kalb, Claudia (June 28, 2004) *Newsweek International* Retrieved Nov 8, 2004 [on line] Available: *http://web7.infotrac.galegroup.com/itw/infomark/*

Legislative Info on the Internet(2004). The Library of Congress. Retrieved Dec. 9, 2004 from http//Thomas.loc.gov

Maine Alzheimer Association (2004) *Legislative Blueprint for Action. Retrieved Dec 14, 2004 from www.mainalz.org/advState legislature.htm*

Namenda Newsletter (2004) *for the Lives Touched by Alzheimer's* Disease. Retrieved Nov. 17, 2004, from www.namenda.com

National Institutes on Health(April, 2004) *Word on Health (on line) available: www.nih.gov/news*

Pitt, Richard (Aug., 2004) *The flue vaccine and you. Retrieved* Dec. 15, 2004. from *http//www.findarticles.com*

Perlmutter, David *ADA Functional Approach* (on line) available: *www.BrainRecovery. com* www.pueblo.gsa.gov /cic_text/helth/alzheim/alzheim.htm

Ralph Walter Richter, 2002. *Alzheimer's Disease* London: Harcourt Ltd. Publishers

Romano, Justin C. (2001) *Neurology Reviews, Vol. 9 No 11 (on line) available: www.neurologyreviews.com*

Charles Schneider's Sons, 1996. *Alzheimer's Disease Dictionary of American History* [on line] Available: *http://galenet.galegroup.com/servlet/histRC/*

Shankle, William Rodman & Amens, Daniel G.(2004) *Preventing Alzheimer's* New York: Penguin Group(USA) Inc.

The Alzheimer Association, New York City Chapter: (2005) Update: Advocacy. Retrieved Feb. 14, 2005 from www.alznyc.org

The Alzheimer's Association (2004) *New York City Chapter Newsletter* Vol. 25 Spring 2004, New York. *www.alznyc.org*

The Alzheimer's Association (2004) *Research and treatment updates and educational meetings* Sept/Oct. 2004, New York

The Alzheimer' Association National Office (on line) available: *www.alz.org*

The Alzheimer's Disease Education & Referral Center (on line) *www.alzheimers.org*

The Alzheimer's Dictionary (on line) available: *www.ahaf.org/alzdis/about/adabout_body.htm*

Mish, Frederick C. (Chief editor)(2001) Webster collegiate dictionary, tenth edition. Massachusetts: Merrian Webster Publisher

Whalley, Lawrence J (2001) *British Journal of Psychiatry* Scotland: University of Aberdeen

Endnotes

[1]   Alzheimer's Association National Office: Ronald and Nancy Reagan Research Institute (1995). Retrieved Nov 7, 2004 from *www.alz.org*

[2]   Kalb, Claudia (June 28, 2001). Newsweek Magazine, p50

[3]   The Alzheimer National Office (2004). Retrieved Oct.19, 2004 from *www.alz.org*

[4]   Biotech Wed Site (2004). Retrieved Oct. 1, 2004 from www.biotechanalyticas.com

[5]   Richter, Ralph Walter (2002) *Alzheimer's Disease London*: Harcourt Ltd. Publishers, page 10,

[6]   The Alzheimer's Dictionary (on line from www.ahaf.org/alzdis/about/adabout_body.htm

[7]   www.npr.org/features/feature.php?wfId=1026693

[8]   Dr Stephen T. Dekosky, (2001) *The Race Against an Alzheimer' Disease Epidemic (as cited on line)www.alz.org/* page 2

[9]   The Alzheimer's Dictionary (on Line from www.ahaf.org/alzdis/about/adabout_body.htm

[10] www.alz.org

[11] Romano, Justin C., (2001) *Neurology Reviews*. Retrieved Oct 5, 2004 from http. www.neurologyreviews.com

[12] Dementia(2004). Retrieved Oct. 29, 2004 from www.dementia.ion.ucl.ac.uk

[13] Webster dictionary, tenth edition (2001)

[14] Webster Collegiate dictionary, tenth edition

[15] Shankle, William Rodman M.S.,M.D., *Preventing Alzheimer's. New York: Penguin Group(USA) Inc.*

[16] Webster Collegiate dictionary, tenth edition

[17] The Alzheimer' National Office (2004). Retrieved Nov 4, 2004 from www.alz.org

[18] Alzheimer Disease Education And Referral Center (2004). Retrieved Nov. 6, 2004from www.alzheimers.org

[19] Ibid Alzheimer Disease Education And Referral Center (2004).Retrieved Nov 9, 2004 from www.alzheimers.org

[20] Alzheimer Disease Education And Referral Center (2004). Retrieved Nov 14, 2004 from www.alxheimers.org

[21] Ibid Alzheimer Disease Education and Referral Center (2004. Retrieved Nov. 16, 2004 from www.alzheimers.org

[22] National Institute Of Aging (2004). Retrieved Dec 2, 2004 from www.alzheimers.org

[23] National Institute Of Aging (2004). Retrieved Dec. 3, 2004 from www.alzheimers.org

[24] Ibid National Instituted Of Aging (2004). Retrieved Dec 5, 2004 from www.alzheimers.org

[25] National Institute of Aging (2004). Retrieved Dec 6, 2004 from www.alzheimers.org

[26] ibid National Institute of Aging (2004). Retrieved Dec.11,2004 fromwww.alzheimers.org

[27] National Instituted of Health (2004). Retrieved Nov. 30, 2004 from www.nih.Gov/news

[28] Alzheimer Association (2004). Retrieved Dec 2, 2004 from www.alz.org/

[29] Alzheimer's Disease Education &Referral Center (2004). Retrieved Nov. 20, 2004 from www.alzheimers.org

[30] Alzheimer Disease Education And Referral Center (2004). Retrieved Dec5, 2004 from wwww.alzheimers.org/pubs/prog00.htm

[31] Consumer Health Science (2004). Retrieved Dec. 3 2004 from www.chsinternational.com/ethdology

[32] Agency For Healthcare Research (2004) Early Alzheimer's Disease. Retrieved Jan. 27 2005 from http://www.ahcpr.gov/clinic/alzcons.htm#head10

[33] Graeber, Manuel & Mehraein (1999) Reanalysis of the First Case of Alzheimer's Disease. Retrieved Dec 22, 2004 from *neuro-www 2.mgh.harvard.ed;u;/adrc_home/history.html*

[34] Ensereink, M(1998)First Alzheimer's diagnosis confirmed. Science 279:2037. Retrieved Dec 22, 2004 from *neuro-www 2.mgh.harvard.ed;u;/adrc_home/history.html*

[35] Ball M. Braak H.(1997) Consensus recommendations for postmortem diagnosis of Alzheimer's disease. Neurobiol Aging, 18 S1-2.Retrieved Jan. 29, 2005 from *neuro-www 2.mgh.harvard.edu/adrc_home/history.html*

[36] Alzheimer's Foundation of America (2004) *Vantage.* Retrieved Jan 29, 2005 from www.alzfdn.org

[37] Romano, Justin C. (2004) The Race Against Alzheimer's Disease Epidemic: Neurology Review 9, 11. Retrieved Jan 29, 2005 from www.Neurologyreview.com

38   The Alzheimer's information Site (2004) The Fischer Center for Alzheimer's. Retrieved Jan. 29, 2005 from www.alzheimers.org

39   Alzheimer's Family Relief Program (2004). Retrieved Dec 23, 2004 from http://www.ahaf.org/afrp/afrp.htm

40   Alzheimer's Family Relief Program (2004). Retrieved Dec 23, 2004 from http://www.ahaf.org/afrp/afrp.htm

41   Alzheimer's Disease: Financial Planning (2004) Retrieved Dec 24, 2004 from http//my.webmd.com

42   Alzheimer's Disease: Financial Planning (2004) Retrieved Dec 24, 2004 from http//my.webmd.com

43   Namenda Newsletter (2004) *Financial, Legal and Insurance Resources. Retrieved Dec 25, 2004 from http://www.namenda.com*

44   Alzheimer's disease (2004) *Managing Your Finances.* Retrieve Dec. 25, 2004 from http://www.alzheimerdisease.com

45   Gilhooly, Mary L *The Dementias, Policy and Management* page 201

46   Alzheimer's Disease Education and Referral Center (2004) Retrieved Jan. 29, 2005 from www.alzheimers.org

47   Hope for the Future through Research (2004). Retrieved Dec 10, 2004 from www.naturaltherapycenter.com/HEALTH%20CONCERNS/alzheimers/

48   Aricept Newsletter (2004) Retrieved Jan. 29, 2005 from www.aricept.com

49   Ibid Aricept Newsletter (2004) Retrieved Dec 10 2004 from www.aricept.com

50   Government Resources(2004). Retrieved Jan 29k 2005 from http://www.pueblo.gsa.gov/cic_text/health/alzheim/alzheim.htm

51   Canadian Study of Heal and Aging (2001) Retrieved Jan 30, 2005 from http://www.cmaj.ca/cgi/content/full/169/6/557

52   Canadian Study of Health and Aging (2001) Retrieved Jan 30, 2005 from http://www.cmaj.ca/cgi/content/full/169/6/557

53   Canadian Census, CBC New in Review, March 2003 page 37

54   Legislative Info on the Internet (2004) The Library of Congress. Retrieved Dec. 9, from http //Thomas.loc.gov

55   Legislative Info on the Internet (2004) The Library of Congress. Retrieved Dec. 9, 2004 from http //Thomas.loc.gov

56   Legislative Info on the Internet (2004) The Library of Congress. Retrieved Dec. 9, 2004 from http//Thomas.loc.gov

57   Whalley, Lawrence J, British Journal of Psychiatry (2001)pg178 (suppl.40) s53-s59

58   Alzheimer's Research: History (2004) Retrieved Jan 20, 2005 from http:www.angelfire.com/oh2/fountainof youth/health.html

59   History of Alzheimer's Disease(2003). Retrieved Oct. 31, 2004 from http://www.eurekalert.org/pub_releases/2003-06/uosf-sla062503.php

60   Alzheimer's Disease: The Costs to U.S. Business (2004) Retrieved Dec.26,2004http://www.solfopro.com/Health/HealthReports/Alzheimers Reportfinalversionpdf#search='alzheimer's:%20social%20costs'

[61] Safran, Dana Gelb (2004) *Social supports as a determinant. Retrieved Dec 9, 2004* (on line)www.findarticles.com

[62] Clinton Earmarks $50 Million for Alzheimer's Research (2000).Retrieved Dec 9, 2004 from archives.cnn.com

[63] Alzheimer Disease: Hope For The Future Through Research (2004). Retrieved Dec 10, 2004 from http:.www.fhma.com

[64] Legislative Initiatives (2004). Retrieved Dec 14, 2004 from http://www.cdc.gov/genomics/about/strategic.htm#action

[65] About Alzheimer's Disease,: Facts, Research(2004). Retrieved Jan 30, 2005 from http://www.ahrq.gov/research/sep96/dept7.htm

[66] Alzheimer's Association Australia (Mar., 02) *Policy Position on Stem Cells.* Retrieved Dec. 12, 2004 from http://www/alzvic.asn.au/stemcells.htm

[67] Pending Stem Cells Research And Legislation (2001). Retrieved Dec 28, 2004 from www.genome.gov

[68] Asbrand, Deborah *Making Political Sense of Stem Cells (2004) Retrieved Dec. 26, 2004 from http://www.technologyreview.com/articles/04/08/wo_asbrand083104.asp?p=0*

[69] Reagan, Michael (June21,2004) *I'm with My Dad on Stem Cell Research.* Retrieved Dec. 28,2004 from http://www.caglecartoons.com

[70] Calacanis, Catherine *Senator Clinton Wants Health Info on Web (2004) from http://telemedicine.weblogsinc.com*

[71] Maine Alzheimer's Association: Legislative Blueprint for Action (2001. Retrieved Dec. 14, 2004www.mainealz.org

[72] Alzheimer's Association and Met life Foundation (Dec 4, 2004) Retrieved Dec 30, 2004 from www.alz.org

[73] Alzheimer's Association and Met life Foundation (Dec 4, 2004) Retrieved Dec 30, 2004 from www.alz.org

[74] The National Endowment For Alzheimer's Research Inc. (2001). Retrieved Jan. 21, 2005 from http://www.memorymatters.org

[75] Rural Information Center: National Foundation (2004). Retrieved from www.nal.usda.gov

[76] New York City Chapter: (2005) Update: Advocacy. Retrieved Feb. 14, 2005 from www.alznyc.org

[77] Pitt, Richard (Aug.,2004) The flue vaccine and you. Retrieved Dec. 15, 2005, from www.findarticles.com

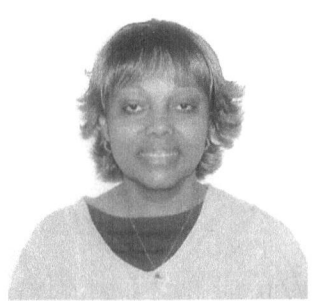 Celestina Akbar, M.P.A (formerly Celestina Bascom) is U.S. Citizen. She was born in Central America. She came with her family to the United State to meet her Uncle, Dr. Chester Holder and his wife. Celestina loved the educational opportunities in the United States. She received a master degree, M.P.A. from C.W. Post, Long Island University. She also graduated from Hunter College and the Borough of Manhattan Community college. She wrote her first book: Alzheimer's Disease: A Growing Health Care Issue Among the Elderly, in fulfillment of her thesis.

www.ingramcontent.com/pod-product-compliance
Lightning Source LLC
Chambersburg PA
CBHW061216280526
45784CB00006B/2513